PROBIOTIC-PACKED BEVERAGES FOR GUT HEALTH

Harness the Power of Fermented Drinks with Simple Recipes for Natural Gut Healing

Lisa A Gentry

TABLE OF CONTENT

5

THE GUT-BRAIN CONNECTION AND WHY FERMENTED DRINKS MATTER

"Did you know that 70% of your immune system resides in your gut?"

This astonishing fact underscores the critical role your digestive system plays in maintaining your overall health. The gut is more than just a site for food digestion—it's a command center that influences your immune function, mental clarity, and even your mood. This is where fermented drinks come into play, acting as powerful tools to nurture and heal your gut.

When you sip on a refreshing glass of kombucha or kefir, you're not just quenching your thirst. You're delivering a potent dose of beneficial bacteria, or probiotics, that can transform your gut health. These "good" bacteria help maintain a balanced gut microbiome, the community of trillions of microorganisms that reside in your digestive tract. From aiding digestion to regulating immune responses, the health of your microbiome directly impacts your overall well-being.

But how exactly does gut health affect your mind and body, and why are fermented drinks such a key part of this equation? To fully understand, we need to dive into the fascinating connection between your gut and brain—often referred to as the "gut-brain axis."

The Gut-Brain Axis: A Two-Way Street

Imagine your gut as a bustling city, constantly communicating with your brain via a network of pathways. This intricate relationship is called the gut-brain axis, a bi-directional communication system that connects the gut and the central nervous system. Signals pass back and forth between the two, influencing everything from how you digest food to how you manage stress.

Here's the fascinating part: much of this communication happens through the gut's microbiome. Your gut bacteria produce neurotransmitters like serotonin and dopamine—chemicals that regulate mood, sleep, and cognitive function. In fact, approximately 90% of the body's serotonin is produced in the gut. This is why an imbalanced gut can lead to mental health issues like anxiety, depression, or brain fog.

Fermented drinks come into the picture as an easy and natural way to restore balance in this complex system. By introducing probiotics into your diet through fermented beverages, you help repopulate your gut with beneficial bacteria. This, in turn, can positively impact both your mental and physical health.

Fermented Drinks: The Secret to a Healthy Microbiome

Fermented drinks like kombucha, kefir, and water kefir are rich in live cultures of probiotics, which are known for their ability to restore and maintain gut flora. Probiotics are the "good guys" of the bacterial world, and they work tirelessly to protect your gut from harmful pathogens, improve digestion, and boost your immune response.

The fermentation process is where the magic happens. Fermentation is the natural transformation of sugars into alcohol or acids by beneficial microorganisms like yeast and bacteria. This process not only preserves the drink but also enhances its nutritional profile. It unlocks beneficial enzymes, B-vitamins, and omega-3 fatty acids, all of which contribute to your health.

When you drink fermented beverages, you're essentially nourishing your body with these powerful probiotics and other nutrients. These drinks offer a simple, accessible way to incorporate gut-friendly bacteria into your diet without complicated supplements or drastic dietary changes.

Let's explore more deeply how fermentation benefits your body.

Why Fermentation Matters: Unlocking the Power of Good Bacteria

Fermentation is an ancient practice, with roots stretching back thousands of years. Cultures around the world have used fermentation as a method to preserve food and drink while enhancing their nutritional value. From sauerkraut in Germany to kimchi in Korea, fermented foods have long been prized for their health benefits. Fermented beverages, such as kombucha and kefir, are no different.

When foods and drinks are fermented, beneficial bacteria and yeast break down sugars and carbohydrates, transforming them into gut-friendly acids and probiotics. The result is a tangy, effervescent drink packed with nutrients that promote digestion, detoxify the body, and strengthen the immune system.

Here are just a few reasons why fermentation is so powerful:

1. **Increases Nutrient Bioavailability:** Fermentation breaks down the anti-nutrients found in many raw ingredients, making vitamins and minerals more readily available for your body to absorb. For instance, the fermentation process can unlock B-vitamins, such as folate and riboflavin, that are essential for energy production and overall health.

2. **Supports Immune Function:** As 70% of the immune system resides in the gut, a healthy microbiome is crucial for immune defense. Fermented drinks introduce good bacteria that enhance immune function by fighting off harmful pathogens and promoting the production of immune cells.

3. **Improves Digestion:** Probiotics help break down food in the digestive tract, making it easier for your body to absorb nutrients. They also reduce bloating, gas, and other digestive discomforts by balancing the bacteria in your gut.

4. **Detoxifies the Body:** Fermented drinks can help cleanse the body by supporting the liver's detoxification processes. Certain probiotic strains are known to bind to and remove toxins from the body, reducing the burden on your liver.

5. **Boosts Mental Clarity:** Remember the gut-brain axis? By improving gut health, fermented drinks can help stabilize mood, reduce anxiety, and enhance mental clarity. Many people report feeling more focused and energized after incorporating probiotic-rich drinks into their diet.

10

Key Ingredients and Tools to Get Started

Before you dive into the recipes for fermented beverages, it's important to gather the right ingredients and tools. Fermenting at home is simple, but it requires attention to detail to ensure safety and success.

Key Ingredients:

1. **Starter Cultures:** To begin fermentation, you'll need a starter culture like a SCOBY (Symbiotic Culture of Bacteria and Yeast) for kombucha or kefir grains for making kefir. These live cultures are the backbone of the fermentation process.

2. **Fresh, Organic Ingredients:** Whether you're using fruits, vegetables, or herbs, opt for organic ingredients to avoid pesticides and harmful chemicals that can disrupt the fermentation process.

3. **Filtered Water:** Many municipal water supplies contain chlorine or other additives that can inhibit fermentation. Always use filtered water to ensure your probiotics thrive.

4. **Natural Sweeteners:** Fermented drinks rely on sugars to fuel the fermentation process. Use natural sweeteners like cane sugar, honey, or fruit juices. The sugar is consumed by the bacteria during fermentation, so the final drink is low in sugar.

Essential Tools:

1. **Glass Jars:** Glass is the ideal vessel for fermenting beverages, as it doesn't react with acidic substances. Large glass jars with tight-fitting lids are a must.

2. **Fermentation Weights:** To keep your ingredients submerged and free from oxygen, you'll need fermentation weights. These ensure a safe, anaerobic environment for fermentation.

3. **Strainers and Funnels:** These are essential for transferring your fermented drinks into bottles once they're ready.

4. **Breathable Covers:** During the initial stages of fermentation, it's important to cover your jars with a breathable cloth or lid to allow gases to escape without letting contaminants in.

How to Safely Ferment Beverages at Home

Fermenting beverages is a safe and rewarding process when done correctly. However, it's important to follow proper hygiene and fermentation practices to avoid contamination or spoilage. Here are some basic guidelines:

1. Cleanliness is Key: Always wash your hands, jars, and tools thoroughly before beginning. Fermentation requires a sterile environment to ensure the right bacteria flourish.
2. Control Temperature: Fermentation works best at temperatures between 68°F and 75°F. Too hot or too cold, and the fermentation process can slow down or stop altogether.
3. Monitor the Process: Check your fermented drinks daily. The fermentation time can vary depending on the temperature and ingredients, so it's important to keep an eye on things.
4. Trust Your Senses: A successful fermentation will result in a tangy, slightly sour taste and a pleasantly effervescent drink. If your drink smells rotten or develops mold, discard it and start again.

!

Chapter 1

KOMBUCHA – THE FIZZ THAT HEALS

"Kombucha, a drink that's been brewed for over 2,000 years, is more than just a trendy health tonic; it's a living, bubbly probiotic powerhouse."

Kombucha, a fermented tea made using a SCOBY (Symbiotic Culture of Bacteria and Yeast), has been cherished for centuries for its potential health benefits, including improving digestion, supporting immune function, and promoting detoxification. This chapter will guide you through the process of brewing your own kombucha at home and show you how to infuse it with exciting flavors, creating a refreshing and nutritious drink that supports your gut health.

Each of these kombucha recipes offers unique flavors and health benefits. Whether you're looking for digestive support, immune-boosting properties, or just a refreshing and healthy drink, kombucha can be a versatile and beneficial addition to your routine!

CLASSIC GREEN TEA KOMBUCHA

Servings: 8 (8-ounce servings)

Prep Time: 30 minutes (plus 7-10 days for fermentation)

Ingredients:

- 8 cups filtered water

- 4 green tea bags (organic preferred)

- 1 cup organic cane sugar

- 1 SCOBY (Symbiotic Culture of Bacteria and Yeast)

- 1 cup kombucha starter liquid (from a previous batch or store-bought unflavored kombucha)

Instructions:

1. **Brew the Tea:** Boil the filtered water, then remove from heat and steep the green tea bags for 10 minutes. Discard the tea bags and stir in the cane sugar until fully dissolved. Let the sweetened tea cool to room temperature.

2. **Prepare the Fermentation Jar:** Pour the cooled tea into a large glass jar, leaving enough space at the top for the SCOBY and starter liquid.

3. **Add the SCOBY and Starter Liquid:** Gently place the SCOBY on top of the tea and pour in the starter liquid. Cover the jar with a breathable cloth (such as a coffee filter or cheesecloth) and secure it with a rubber band.

4. **Fermentation:** Let the jar sit in a warm, dark place for 7-10 days. Taste the kombucha after day 7 and let it ferment longer if you prefer a tangier flavor.

5. **Bottle and Second Ferment (Optional):** After fermentation, remove the SCOBY and 1 cup of kombucha (to use as starter liquid for your next batch). Bottle the kombucha in airtight glass bottles. For carbonation, let the bottles sit for 2-3 more days at room temperature before refrigerating.

Tips:

- Always use non-metal utensils when handling the SCOBY to avoid contamination.

- The longer kombucha ferments, the less sweet and more tart it becomes.

Nutritional Values (Per 8-ounce serving):

- Calories: 30

- Probiotics: High

- Sugar: 3g (varies with fermentation time)

- Antioxidants: High, due to green tea

GINGER-LEMON KOMBUCHA FOR IMMUNITY

Servings: 8 (8-ounce servings)

Prep Time: 35 minutes (plus 7-10 days for fermentation)

Ingredients:

- 8 cups filtered water

- 4 black tea bags

- 1 cup organic cane sugar

- 1 SCOBY

- 1 cup kombucha starter liquid

- 2-inch piece fresh ginger, sliced

- Juice of 2 lemons

- 1 tablespoon raw honey (optional)

Instructions:

1. **Prepare the Tea:** Brew the black tea in boiled water and dissolve the sugar. Allow it to cool to room temperature.

2. **Fermentation:** Add the cooled tea, SCOBY, and starter liquid to a large jar, cover with a cloth, and let ferment for 7-10 days.

3. **Flavoring:** After the first fermentation, remove the SCOBY. Pour the kombucha into bottles, adding ginger slices and lemon juice to each bottle. Seal tightly and ferment for an additional 2-3 days for natural carbonation.

4. **Enjoy:** After the second fermentation, refrigerate and enjoy chilled.

Tips:

- Ginger promotes digestion and helps reduce inflammation.

- Lemon juice boosts vitamin C, perfect for immune support.

Nutritional Values (Per 8-ounce serving):

- Calories: 40

- Probiotics: High

- Sugar: 5g (varies with fermentation time)

- Vitamin C: 20mg (from lemon juice)

BERRY BLAST KOMBUCHA WITH ANTIOXIDANTS

Servings: 8 (8-ounce servings)

Prep Time: 30 minutes (plus 7-10 days for fermentation)

Ingredients:

- 8 cups filtered water

- 4 oolong tea bags

- 1 cup organic cane sugar

- 1 SCOBY

- 1 cup kombucha starter liquid

- 1/2 cup mixed berries (strawberries, blueberries, raspberries)

Instructions:

1. **Brew Tea:** Steep the oolong tea and dissolve the sugar. Cool to room temperature.

2. **Fermentation:** Add the tea, SCOBY, and starter liquid to a jar and ferment for 7-10 days.

3. **Flavoring:** After the first fermentation, remove the SCOBY and add the kombucha to bottles with mixed berries. Ferment for 2-3 days more to infuse the berry flavor.

4. **Chill and Serve:** Once carbonated, refrigerate and enjoy.

Tips:

- Berries add a boost of antioxidants to fight free radicals.

- You can mash the berries slightly for more intense flavor.

Nutritional Values (Per 8-ounce serving):

- Calories: 50

- Probiotics: High

- Sugar: 6g

- Antioxidants: High

TROPICAL PINEAPPLE-MANGO KOMBUCHA

Servings: 8 (8-ounce servings)

Prep Time: 30 minutes (plus 7-10 days for fermentation)

Ingredients:

- 8 cups filtered water

- 4 white tea bags

- 1 cup organic cane sugar

- 1 SCOBY

- 1 cup kombucha starter liquid

- 1/2 cup fresh pineapple, chopped

- 1/2 cup fresh mango, chopped

Instructions:

1. **Prepare Tea:** Brew white tea and dissolve sugar, then cool.

2. **Fermentation:** Add the tea, SCOBY, and starter liquid to your jar and ferment for 7-10 days.

3. **Second Fermentation:** After removing the SCOBY, bottle the kombucha with pineapple and mango. Let it ferment for 2-3 days for flavor infusion.

4. **Serve:** Once carbonated, chill and enjoy.

Tips:

- Tropical fruits like pineapple and mango give a vitamin C boost.

- Be sure to strain the kombucha before drinking if you prefer no fruit pulp.

Nutritional Values (Per 8-ounce serving):

- Calories: 55

- Probiotics: High

- Sugar: 7g

- Vitamin C: 30mg

SPICED APPLE CINNAMON KOMBUCHA

Servings: 8 (8-ounce servings)

Prep Time: 30 minutes (plus 7-10 days for fermentation)

Ingredients:

- 8 cups filtered water

- 4 black tea bags

- 1 cup organic cane sugar

- 1 SCOBY

- 1 cup kombucha starter liquid

- 1 cup apple cider

- 1 cinnamon stick

- 1/2 teaspoon ground cloves

Instructions:

1. **Brew Tea:** Brew black tea and dissolve sugar. Cool the mixture.

2. **Fermentation:** Add tea, SCOBY, and starter liquid, and ferment for 7-10 days.

3. **Second Fermentation:** Bottle the kombucha with apple cider, cinnamon stick, and cloves. Let it ferment for 2-3 days to infuse flavors.

4. **Chill and Enjoy:** After carbonating, refrigerate and serve cold.

Tips:

- Perfect for fall, this kombucha has a comforting spice flavor.

- Try adding a splash of fresh apple juice before serving for extra sweetness.

Nutritional Values (Per 8-ounce serving):

- Calories: 60

- Probiotics: High

- Sugar: 6g

- Fiber: Low, but the cinnamon adds digestive benefits.

LAVENDER & CHAMOMILE KOMBUCHA FOR STRESS RELIEF

Servings: 8 (8-ounce servings)

Prep Time: 30 minutes (plus 7-10 days for fermentation)

Ingredients:

- 8 cups filtered water

- 4 green tea bags

- 1 cup organic cane sugar

- 1 SCOBY

- 1 cup kombucha starter liquid

- 1 tablespoon dried lavender

- 1 tablespoon dried chamomile flowers

Instructions:

1. **Brew Tea:** Steep green tea, dissolve sugar, and cool.

2. **Fermentation:** Add the tea, SCOBY, and starter liquid to a jar and ferment for 7-10 days.

3. **Flavoring:** Remove the SCOBY, then bottle the kombucha with lavender and chamomile. Let it ferment for 2-3 more days.

4. **Strain and Chill:** Strain out the flowers and refrigerate.

Tips:

- Both lavender and chamomile are known for their calming properties, making this a perfect evening kombucha.

- Pair with a relaxing activity like yoga or meditation.

Nutritional Values (Per 8-ounce serving):

- Calories: 35

- Probiotics: High

- Sugar: 4g

- Herbal Benefits: Helps reduce anxiety and promotes better sleep.

TURMERIC KOMBUCHA FOR ANTI-INFLAMMATION

Servings: 8 (8-ounce servings)

Prep Time: 30 minutes (plus 7-10 days for fermentation)

Ingredients:

- 8 cups filtered water

- 4 black tea bags

- 1 cup organic cane sugar

- 1 SCOBY

- 1 cup kombucha starter liquid

- 1 teaspoon ground turmeric

- 1/2 teaspoon black pepper (to increase absorption)

Instructions:

1. **Prepare Tea:** Brew black tea and dissolve sugar, then cool.

2. **Fermentation:** Add the tea, SCOBY, and starter liquid, and let it ferment for 7-10 days.

3. **Second Fermentation:** Remove the SCOBY, then bottle the kombucha with turmeric and black pepper. Let it ferment for 2-3 days for extra flavor.

4. **Chill:** After carbonation, refrigerate and enjoy.

Tips:

- Turmeric has potent anti-inflammatory properties and works best when paired with black pepper to enhance absorption.

- This kombucha is great post-workout to reduce muscle soreness.

Nutritional Values (Per 8-ounce serving):

- Calories: 40

- Probiotics: High

- Sugar: 5g

- Anti-inflammatory Compounds: Curcumin from turmeri

WATERMELON MINT KOMBUCHA – A REFRESHING SUMMER TREAT

Servings: 8 (8-ounce servings)

Prep Time: 30 minutes (plus 7-10 days for fermentation)

Ingredients:

- 8 cups filtered water
- 4 white tea bags
- 1 cup organic cane sugar
- 1 SCOBY
- 1 cup kombucha starter liquid
- 1/2 cup fresh watermelon chunks
- 10-12 fresh mint leaves

Instructions:

1. **Brew Tea:** Brew white tea and dissolve the sugar. Cool to room temperature.

2. **Fermentation:** Add tea, SCOBY, and starter liquid to a jar and ferment for 7-10 days.

3. **Flavoring:** After the first fermentation, bottle the kombucha with watermelon and mint leaves. Let it ferment for 2-3 days for extra flavor and fizz.

4. **Serve:** After carbonation, strain, chill, and serve cold.

Tips:

- Perfect for hot summer days, the watermelon adds hydration while the mint provides a cooling sensation.

- Strain the watermelon and mint out if you prefer a clearer drink.

Nutritional Values (Per 8-ounce serving):

- Calories: 40

- Probiotics: High

- Sugar: 5g

- Hydration: Watermelon provides electrolytes and hydration.

Chapter 2

KEFIR – TANGY AND TUMMY-FRIENDLY

"Kefir contains over 30 strains of beneficial bacteria and yeasts—making it one of the most potent probiotics on the planet."

Kefir is a fermented milk drink, but in this chapter, we'll also explore plant-based alternatives like coconut and almond kefir. These easy-to-make drinks are loaded with probiotics to aid digestion and improve gut health.

These kefir recipes not only provide delicious ways to incorporate probiotics into your diet but also promote gut health, making them a fantastic addition to your daily routine. Enjoy experimenting with these delightful concoctions!

CLASSIC MILK KEFIR WITH HONEY

Servings: 4 (1-cup servings)

Prep Time: 10 minutes (plus fermentation time: 24 hours)

Ingredients:

- 4 cups whole milk (or any milk of your choice)

- 1/4 cup milk kefir grains

- 2 tablespoons honey (or to taste)

Instructions:

1. **Combine Ingredients:** In a clean glass jar, combine the milk and milk kefir grains. Stir gently with a wooden spoon to mix.

2. **Fermentation:** Cover the jar with a breathable cloth (like cheesecloth) and secure it with a rubber band. Let it sit at room temperature for 24 hours, away from direct sunlight.

3. **Strain:** After 24 hours, the mixture should be thickened and tangy. Strain the kefir through a fine mesh sieve into a clean jar, discarding the grains (or reserving them for future batches).

4. **Add Honey:** Stir in the honey until fully dissolved. You can also blend it for a smoother texture.

5. **Chill and Serve:** Refrigerate for a few hours before serving. Enjoy it cold!

Tips:

- For a thicker kefir, let it ferment for an additional 12-24 hours.

- You can use the reserved kefir grains to make more batches or give them to friends.

Nutritional Values (Per 1-cup serving):

- Calories: 150

- Protein: 8g

- Fat: 8g

- Carbohydrates: 12g

- Sugar: 6g (natural sugars from milk)

COCONUT KEFIR FOR DAIRY-FREE GUT HEALING

Servings: 4 (1-cup servings)

Prep Time: 10 minutes (plus fermentation time: 24-48 hours)

Ingredients:

- 4 cups coconut milk (canned or carton)

- 1/4 cup water kefir grains (or coconut kefir starter)

- 1-2 tablespoons maple syrup (optional, for sweetness)

Instructions:

1. **Mix Ingredients:** In a clean glass jar, mix the coconut milk and water kefir grains (or starter). Stir gently.

2. **Fermentation:** Cover with a breathable cloth and secure it. Let it sit at room temperature for 24-48 hours, depending on desired tanginess.

3. **Strain:** After fermentation, strain the kefir through a fine mesh sieve into a clean jar. Discard the grains or save them for future use.

4. **Sweeten (Optional):** Stir in maple syrup if desired.

5. **Chill and Serve:** Refrigerate for a few hours before serving.

Tips:

- Use full-fat coconut milk for a creamier texture.

- Coconut kefir can also be blended with fruit for a delicious smoothie.

Nutritional Values (Per 1-cup serving):

- Calories: 150 - Protein: 1g - Fat: 15g

- Carbohydrates: 6g

- Sugar: 3g (if maple syrup is added) - Probiotics: High (beneficial yeasts and bacteria)

STRAWBERRY VANILLA KEFIR SMOOTHIE

Servings: 2 (1-cup servings)

Prep Time: 5 minutes

Ingredients:

- 1 cup classic milk kefir (or coconut kefir)

- 1 cup fresh strawberries (or frozen)

- 1 banana

- 1 teaspoon pure vanilla extract

- 1 tablespoon honey or maple syrup (optional)

Instructions:

1. **Blend Ingredients:** In a blender, combine the kefir, strawberries, banana, vanilla extract, and honey or maple syrup.

2. **Blend** Until Smooth: Blend until creamy and smooth.

3. **Serve Immediately:** Pour into glasses and enjoy!

Tips:

- Add a handful of spinach or kale for an extra nutrient boost.

- This smoothie is great for breakfast or as a post-workout snack.

Nutritional Values (Per 1-cup serving):

- Calories: 120

- Protein: 6g

- Fat: 2g

- Carbohydrates: 24g

- Sugar: 12g

- Probiotics: High

CHIA SEED KEFIR PUDDING – A NUTRIENT-PACKED BREAKFAST

Servings: 4 (1-cup servings)

Prep Time: 10 minutes (plus soaking time: 4 hours or overnight)

Ingredients:

- 2 cups milk kefir (or coconut kefir)

- 1/2 cup chia seeds

- 1 tablespoon honey or maple syrup (optional)

- 1 teaspoon vanilla extract

- Fresh fruits for topping (e.g., berries, banana slices)

Instructions:

1. **Combine Ingredients:** In a bowl, whisk together kefir, chia seeds, honey, and vanilla extract until combined.

2. **Soak:** Cover and refrigerate for at least 4 hours or overnight until the chia seeds expand and thicken the mixture.

3. **Serve:** Spoon into bowls and top with fresh fruits before serving

Tips:

- Stir the mixture halfway through the soaking time for even thickness.

- Chia seed pudding can be stored in the refrigerator for up to 5 days.

Nutritional Values (Per 1-cup serving):

- Calories: 180

- Protein: 7g

- Fat: 6g

- Carbohydrates: 22g

- Sugar: 5g - Probiotics: High

KEFIR LEMONADE – A TANGY TWIST ON A SUMMER FAVORITE

Servings: 4 (1-cup servings)

Prep Time: 10 minutes (plus fermentation time: 2-3 hours)

Ingredients:

- 2 cups milk kefir (or coconut kefir)

- 1/2 cup fresh lemon juice

- 1/4 cup honey or agave syrup (adjust to taste)

- 2 cups water

- Lemon slices and mint for garnish

Instructions:

1. Mix Ingredients: In a large pitcher, combine the kefir, lemon juice, honey, and water. Stir well until the honey dissolves.

2. Fermentation (Optional): If you want a tangier flavor, let the mixture sit at room temperature for 2-3 hours before chilling.

3. Serve: Pour over ice and garnish with lemon slices and mint.

Tips:

- Adjust the sweetness by adding more or less honey.

- This drink is perfect for summer gatherings.

Nutritional Values (Per 1-cup serving):

- Calories: 90

- Protein: 4g

- Fat: 2g

- Carbohydrates: 16g

- Sugar: 10g - Probiotics: High

ALMOND KEFIR FOR VEGAN PROBIOTIC BOOST

Servings: 4 (1-cup servings)

Prep Time: 10 minutes (plus fermentation time: 24-48 hours)

Ingredients:

- 4 cups almond milk (unsweetened)

- 1/4 cup water kefir grains (or a vegan kefir starter)

- 1-2 tablespoons maple syrup (optional)

Instructions:

1. Combine Ingredients: In a glass jar, mix almond milk and water kefir grains (or starter).

2. Fermentation: Cover with a breathable cloth and let sit at room temperature for 24-48 hours.

3. Strain: Strain the kefir into a clean jar, discarding the grains or saving for future use.

4. Sweeten (Optional): Stir in maple syrup if desired.

5. Chill and Serve: Refrigerate before serving.

Tips:

- Experiment with flavored almond milk for different tastes.

- Use a high-quality almond milk for the best results.

Nutritional Values (Per 1-cup serving):

- Calories: 60

- Protein: 2g

- Fat: 3g

- Carbohydrates: 6g

- Sugar: 1g - Probiotics: High

BLUEBERRY BANANA KEFIR SMOOTHIE

Servings: 2 (1-cup servings)

Prep Time: 5 minutes

Ingredients:

- 1 cup milk kefir (or coconut kefir)

- 1 banana

- 1 cup blueberries (fresh or frozen)

- 1 tablespoon honey or maple syrup (optional)

- 1 tablespoon flaxseeds (optional for extra fiber)

Instructions:

1. **Blend Ingredients:** In a blender, combine kefir, banana, blueberries, honey, and flaxseeds.

2. **Blend Until Smooth:** Blend until creamy and smooth.

3. **Serve Immediately:** Pour into glasses and enjoy!

Tips:

- Add a handful of spinach for a green smoothie boost.

- This smoothie is an excellent way to start your day.

Nutritional Values (Per 1-cup serving):

- Calories: 120

- Protein: 5g

- Fat: 2g

- Carbohydrates: 26g

- Sugar: 12g - Probiotics: High

KEFIR ICED COFFEE – AN ENERGIZING GUT-FRIENDLY DRINK

Servings: 2 (1-cup servings)

Prep Time: 5 minutes

Ingredients:

- 1 cup brewed coffee (cooled)

- 1 cup milk kefir (or coconut kefir)

- 1 tablespoon cocoa powder (optional)

- 1 tablespoon sweetener (honey, sugar, or syrup)

- Ice cubes

Instructions:

1. Mix Ingredients: In a large glass, combine the cooled coffee, kefir, cocoa powder, and sweetener.

2. Stir: Mix well until combined.

3. Serve: Fill two glasses with ice cubes and pour the mixture over the ice. Stir gently.

Tips:

- For a mocha flavor, increase the cocoa powder.

- This drink can be a great afternoon pick-me-up.

Nutritional Values (Per 1-cup serving):

- Calories: 100

- Protein: 6g

- Fat: 3g

- Carbohydrates: 12g

- Sugar: 5g - Probiotics: High

Chapter 3

LACTO-FERMENTED LEMONADES – CITRUS WITH A PROBIOTIC KICK

"Lemonade doesn't just quench your thirst, it can also fuel your gut with beneficial bacteria when fermented."

In this chapter, we reimagine traditional lemonade using lacto-fermentation to create tangy, probiotic-packed beverages. These delicious lemonades not only satisfy your thirst but also promote gut health, thanks to the beneficial bacteria produced during fermentation. With a variety of flavors and health benefits, these refreshing drinks are perfect for any occasion!

These lacto-fermented lemonade recipes provide a delightful way to stay hydrated while nourishing your gut with beneficial probiotics. Enjoy these tangy beverages throughout the year for a refreshing and healthful treat!

CLASSIC LACTO-FERMENTED LEMONADE

Servings: 6 (1-cup servings)

Prep Time: 10 minutes (plus fermentation time: 2-3 days)

Ingredients:

- 1 cup fresh lemon juice (about 4-6 lemons)

- 1/2 cup honey or cane sugar

- 4 cups filtered water

- 1/4 cup whey (from yogurt) or 2 tablespoons sea salt

- Optional: lemon slices for garnish

Instructions:

1. **Dissolve Sweetener:** In a large mixing bowl, combine lemon juice and honey (or sugar). Stir until fully dissolved.

2. **Add Water:** Pour in the filtered water and mix well.

3. **Incorporate Whey or Salt:** Stir in the whey (or sea salt) to introduce beneficial bacteria.

4. **Ferment:** Transfer the mixture to a clean glass jar or fermenting vessel, leaving about an inch of headspace. Seal it loosely to allow gas to escape.

5. **Fermentation:** Place the jar in a cool, dark place for 2-3 days. Check daily; it should become tangy and slightly fizzy.

6. **Chill and Serve:** Once fermented to your liking, refrigerate and enjoy chilled. Garnish with lemon slices if desired.

Tips:

- Use organic lemons for the best flavor and health benefits

Nutritional Values (Per 1-cup serving):

- Calories: 90 - Protein: 0g

- Fat: 0g - Carbohydrates: 22g

- Sugar: 20g - Probiotics: High

GINGER-TURMERIC LEMONADE FOR INFLAMMATION RELIEF

Servings: 6 (1-cup servings)

Prep Time: 15 minutes (plus fermentation time: 2-3 days)

Ingredients:

- 1 cup fresh lemon juice

- 1/4 cup grated fresh ginger

- 1 tablespoon grated fresh turmeric (or 1 teaspoon turmeric powder)

- 1/2 cup honey or agave syrup

- 4 cups filtered water

- 1/4 cup whey (or 2 tablespoons sea salt)

Instructions:

1. **Prepare Ingredients**: In a large bowl, combine lemon juice, grated ginger, grated turmeric, and honey. Stir until the honey dissolves.

2. **Add Water**: Mix in the filtered water.

3. **Incorporate Whey or Salt**: Stir in the whey (or sea salt).

4. **Ferment**: Pour the mixture into a glass jar, sealing it loosely. Allow it to ferment in a cool, dark place for 2-3 days.

5. **Chill and Serve**: Refrigerate once fermented. Serve chilled, stirring before pouring.

Tips:

- For a spicier kick, increase the ginger quantity.

- Use a strainer to remove ginger and turmeric pieces before serving, if preferred.

Nutritional Values (Per 1-cup serving):

- Calories: 95 - Protein: 0g

- Fat: 0g - Carbohydrates: 24g

- Sugar: 20g - Probiotics: High

34

RASPBERRY BASIL LACTO-FERMENTED LEMONADE

Servings: 6 (1-cup servings)

Prep Time: 15 minutes (plus fermentation time: 2-3 days)

Ingredients:

- 1 cup fresh lemon juice

- 1 cup fresh raspberries (or frozen)

- 1/2 cup honey or sugar

- 4 cups filtered water

- 1/4 cup fresh basil leaves, chopped

- 1/4 cup whey (or 2 tablespoons sea salt)

Instructions:

1. **Muddle Raspberries**: In a large bowl, muddle the raspberries to release their juices.

2. **Combine Ingredients**: Add lemon juice, honey, and water to the bowl. Stir until honey dissolves.

3. **Add Basil and Whey/Salt**: Mix in chopped basil and whey (or sea salt).

4. **Ferment**: Transfer to a glass jar and seal loosely. Let ferment for 2-3 days.

5. **Strain and Serve**: After fermentation, strain out the raspberry seeds and basil leaves. Chill before serving.

Tips:

- Garnish with whole raspberries and basil leaves for presentation.

- Use a fine mesh sieve for straining to get a smooth texture.

Nutritional Values (Per 1-cup serving):

- Calories: 90

- Protein: 0g

- Fat: 0g

- Carbohydrates: 23g

- Sugar: 20g - Probiotics: High

LAVENDER HONEY LEMONADE FOR RELAXATION

Servings: 6 (1-cup servings)

Prep Time: 10 minutes (plus fermentation time: 2-3 days)

Ingredients:

- 1 cup fresh lemon juice

- 1/4 cup dried lavender flowers

- 1/2 cup honey

- 4 cups filtered water

- 1/4 cup whey (or 2 tablespoons sea salt)

Instructions:

1. **Infuse Lavender:** In a saucepan, bring 2 cups of water to a boil. Remove from heat, add dried lavender, and steep for 10-15 minutes. Strain and cool.

2. **Mix Ingredients:** In a large bowl, combine lemon juice, lavender infusion, honey, and the remaining 2 cups of filtered water.

3. **Incorporate Whey or Salt:** Stir in the whey (or sea salt).

4. **Ferment:** Pour into a glass jar, sealing loosely, and let ferment for 2-3 days.

5. **Chill and Serve:** Once fermented, refrigerate and enjoy chilled.

Tips:

- Adjust lavender amount for more or less floral flavor.

- This lemonade is great for calming evenings.

Nutritional Values (Per 1-cup serving):

- Calories: 85

- Protein: 0g

- Fat: 0g

- Carbohydrates: 22g

- Sugar: 20g - Probiotics: High

SPICY JALAPEÑO LIME LEMONADE – A PROBIOTIC KICK WITH HEAT

Servings: 6 (1-cup servings)

Prep Time: 15 minutes (plus fermentation time: 2-3 days)

Ingredients:

- 1 cup fresh lemon juice

- 1/2 cup fresh lime juice

- 1-2 fresh jalapeños, sliced (adjust to taste)

- 1/2 cup honey or agave syrup

- 4 cups filtered water

- 1/4 cup whey (or 2 tablespoons sea salt)

Instructions:

1. **Combine Ingredients:** In a large bowl, mix lemon juice, lime juice, sliced jalapeños, and honey until honey dissolves.

2. **Add Water:** Stir in the filtered water.

3. **Incorporate Whey or Salt:** Add whey (or sea salt) and mix well.

4. **Ferment:** Pour the mixture into a glass jar, sealing loosely, and let ferment for 2-3 days.

5. **Chill and Serve:** Once fermented, strain out the jalapeños if desired. Chill before serving.

Tips:

- Use gloves when handling jalapeños to avoid irritation.

- For a smoky flavor, try adding a pinch of smoked paprika.

Nutritional Values (Per 1-cup serving):

- Calories: 90

- Protein: 0g

- Fat: 0g

- Carbohydrates: 22g

- Sugar: 20g - Probiotics: High

ORANGE AND THYME LACTO LEMONADE

Servings: 6 (1-cup servings)

Prep Time: 10 minutes (plus fermentation time: 2-3 days)

Ingredients:

- 1 cup fresh lemon juice

- 1 cup fresh orange juice

- 1/4 cup fresh thyme leaves

- 1/2 cup honey or agave syrup

- 4 cups filtered water

- 1/4 cup whey (or 2 tablespoons sea salt

) **Instructions:**

1. Mix Juices: In a large bowl, combine lemon juice, orange juice, thyme leaves, and honey. Stir until honey dissolves.

2. Add Water: Pour in the filtered water and mix well.

3. Incorporate Whey or Salt: Stir in whey (or sea salt).

4. Ferment: Transfer to a glass jar, sealing loosely, and allow to ferment for 2-3 days.

5. Chill and Serve: After fermentation, strain out thyme leaves. Refrigerate before serving.

Tips:

- Garnish with fresh thyme sprigs for an elegant touch.

- Experiment with different citrus combinations for unique flavors.

Nutritional Values (Per 1-c up serving):

- Calories: 90

- Protein: 0g

- Fat: 0g

- Carbohydrates: 22g

- Sugar: 20g - Probiotics: High

CUCUMBER MINT LEMONADE – HYDRATION AND GUT SUPPORT

Servings: 6 (1-cup servings)

Prep Time: 10 minutes (plus fermentation time: 2-3 days)

Ingredients:

- 1 cup fresh lemon juice
- 1 medium cucumber, sliced
- 1/4 cup fresh mint leaves
- 1/2 cup honey or agave syrup
- 4 cups filtered water
- 1/4 cup whey (or 2 tablespoons sea salt)

Instructions:

1. **Combine Ingredients:** In a large bowl, mix lemon juice, cucumber slices, mint leaves, and honey until honey dissolves.

2. **Add Water:** Stir in the filtered water.

3. **Incorporate Whey or Salt:** Add whey (or sea salt) and mix well.

4. **Ferment:** Pour the mixture into a glass jar, sealing loosely, and let ferment for 2-3 days.

5. **Chill and Serve:** After fermentation, strain out cucumber and mint if desired. Serve chilled.

Tips:

- This refreshing drink is perfect for summer.
- Add additional cucumber slices for garnish.

Nutritional Values (Per 1-cup serving):

- Calories: 85
- Protein: 0g
- Fat: 0g
- Carbohydrates: 21g
- Sugar: 20g - Probiotics: High

LACTO-FERMENTED LEMONADE SLUSHIES – PERFECT FOR HOT DAYS

Servings: 4 (1-cup servings)

Prep Time: 10 minutes (plus fermentation time: 2-3 days)

Ingredients:

- 2 cups classic lacto-fermented lemonade (see recipe 1)

- 1 cup ice cubes

- Optional: fresh fruit or herbs for garnish

Instructions:

1. **Prepare Lemonade:** Follow the classic lacto-fermented lemonade recipe and allow it to ferment.

2. **Blend:** In a blender, combine the fermented lemonade and ice cubes. Blend until smooth and slushy.

3. **Serve:** Pour into glasses and garnish with fresh fruit or herbs if desired.

Tips:

- Experiment with different garnishes like berries or mint leaves.

- This slushie makes a great summer party drink.

Nutritional Values (Per 1-cup serving):

- Calories: 60

- Protein: 0g

- Fat: 0g

- Carbohydrates: 15g

- Sugar: 14g - Probiotics: High

Chapter 4

FERMENTED HERBAL TEAS – SIP YOUR WAY TO A BALANCED GUT

"Did you know that herbs like chamomile, peppermint, and rooibos can be fermented to create drinks that soothe the gut and promote digestion?"

Herbal teas are known for their calming properties, but when fermented, they deliver even more health benefits. This chapter delves into fermented herbal infusions that boost gut health and flavor. Get ready to brew up a collection of delightful herbal teas that are not only delicious but also enhance your well-being.

These recipes not only highlight the delightful flavors of herbal teas but also harness the power of fermentation to promote gut health. Enjoy experimenting with these delicious brews, each offering unique benefits and a refreshing twist on traditional herbal infusions!

FERMENTED CHAMOMILE TEA FOR SLEEP AND DIGESTION

Servings: 4 (1-cup servings)

Prep Time: 15 minutes (plus fermentation time: 2-3 days)

Ingredients:

- 4 cups water

- 4 chamomile tea bags (or 4 tablespoons dried chamomile flowers)

- 1/4 cup honey or agave syrup

- 1/4 cup whey (or 2 tablespoons sea salt)

- Optional: 1 teaspoon vanilla extract (for added flavor)

Instructions:

1. **Boil Water:** Bring the water to a boil in a saucepan.

2. **Steep Tea:** Remove from heat, add the chamomile tea bags, and steep for 10 minutes. Remove the bags and let the tea cool to room temperature.

3. **Sweeten:** Stir in honey or agave syrup until dissolved.

4. **Add Culture:** Once cooled, add whey or sea salt, and mix well.

5. **Ferment:** Pour the mixture into a glass jar, sealing it loosely. Let it ferment at room temperature for 2-3 days, tasting daily until desired sourness is achieved.

6. **Store:** Once fermented, refrigerate and serve chilled.

Tips:

- For a stronger flavor, steep the tea longer.

- Enjoy hot or cold; both versions are soothing.

Nutritional Values (Per 1-cup serving):

- Calories: 65 - Protein: 0g

- Fat: 0g - Carbohydrates: 17g

- Sugar: 16g - Probiotics: High

PEPPERMINT KOMBUCHA FOR FRESHNESS AND GUT HEALING

Servings: 4 (1-cup servings)

Prep Time: 20 minutes (plus fermentation time: 7-14 days)

Ingredients:

- 4 cups water

- 1 cup sugar

- 4 bags black tea (or 4 tablespoons loose-leaf)

- 1 cup starter kombucha (from a previous batch)

- 1/4 cup fresh peppermint leaves (or 2-3 bags peppermint tea)

- Optional: 1 lemon, sliced (for added zest)

Instructions:

1. **Prepare Sweet Tea:** Boil water, stir in sugar until dissolved, and add tea bags. Steep for 10 minutes and let cool to room temperature.

2. **Combine Ingredients:** In a large glass jar, combine the sweet tea, starter kombucha, and fresh peppermint.

3. **Ferment:** Cover the jar with a cloth secured with a rubber band. Let it ferment for 7-14 days, tasting every few days until you reach your preferred level of tanginess.

4. **Bottle:** Once ready, strain the mixture into bottles, leaving some sediment behind.

5. **Store:** Seal bottles and refrigerate. Enjoy chilled.

Tips:

- Use a SCOBY (Symbiotic Culture Of Bacteria and Yeast) to kickstart the fermentation.

Nutritional Values (Per 1-cup serving):

- Calories: 40 - Protein: 0g

- Fat: 0g - Carbohydrates: 10g

- Sugar: 9g - Probiotics: High

HIBISCUS GINGER FERMENTED ICED TEA – RICH IN ANTIOXIDANTS

Servings: 4 (1-cup servings)

Prep Time: 15 minutes (plus fermentation time: 2-3 days)

Ingredients:

- 4 cups water

- 1/4 cup dried hibiscus flowers

- 2 tablespoons grated fresh ginger

- 1/4 cup honey or maple syrup

- 1/4 cup whey (or 2 tablespoons sea salt)

Instructions:

1. **Boil Water:** Bring water to a boil.

2. **Steep Ingredients:** Add hibiscus flowers and ginger to boiling water. Remove from heat and steep for 10 minutes. Strain and let cool to room temperature.

3. **Sweeten:** Stir in honey or maple syrup until dissolved.

4. **Add Culture:** Mix in whey or sea salt.

5. **Ferment:** Pour the mixture into a glass jar and ferment at room temperature for 2-3 days.

6. **Serve:** Once fermented, strain and serve chilled over ice.

Tips:

- Garnish with fresh mint leaves for an added burst of flavor.

- Hibiscus tea is naturally tart; adjust sweetness to your taste.

Nutritional Values (Per 1-cup serving):

- Calories: 70

- Protein: 0g

- Fat: 0g - Carbohydrates: 18g- Sugar: 17g

- Probiotics: High

ROOIBOS AND VANILLA FERMENTED TEA – CAFFEINE-FREE AND GUT-FRIENDLY

Servings: 4 (1-cup servings)

Prep Time: 15 minutes (plus fermentation time: 2-3 days)

Ingredients:

- 4 cups water

- 4 rooibos tea bags (or 4 tablespoons loose-leaf rooibos)

- 1/4 cup honey or agave syrup

- 1 teaspoon vanilla extract

- 1/4 cup whey (or 2 tablespoons sea salt)

Instructions:

1. **Boil Water:** Bring water to a boil.

2. **Steep Tea:** Remove from heat, add rooibos tea bags, and steep for 10 minutes. Remove tea bags and let cool.

3. **Sweeten:** Stir in honey or agave syrup and vanilla extract until dissolved.

4. **Add Culture:** Mix in whey or sea salt.

5. **Ferment:** Pour into a glass jar, seal loosely, and let it ferment at room temperature for 2-3 days.

6. **Store and Serve:** Once fermented, refrigerate and enjoy chilled.

Tips:

- Rooibos is naturally sweet; adjust sweetness as desired.

- This tea can be enjoyed warm or cold.

Nutritional Values (Per 1-cup serving):

- Calories: 65

- Protein: 0g

- Fat: 0g - Carbohydrates: 17g

- Sugar: 16g - Probiotics: High

FERMENTED GREEN TEA WITH LEMONGRASS

Servings: 4 (1-cup servings)

Prep Time: 15 minutes (plus fermentation time: 2-3 days)

Ingredients:

- 4 cups water

- 4 green tea bags (or 4 tablespoons loose-leaf green tea)

- 1/4 cup honey or agave syrup

- 1/2 cup fresh lemongrass, chopped

- 1/4 cup whey (or 2 tablespoons sea salt)

Instructions:

1. **Boil Water:** Bring water to a boil.

2. **Steep Tea and Lemongrass:** Add tea bags and lemongrass to boiling water. Steep for 5 minutes, then remove tea bags and let cool.

3. **Sweeten:** Stir in honey or agave syrup until dissolved.

4. **Add Culture:** Mix in whey or sea salt.

5. **Ferment:** Pour into a glass jar and ferment at room temperature for 2-3 days.

6. **Serve:** Once ready, strain and enjoy chilled.

Tips:

- This tea is refreshing and great for hot weather.

- Use a citrus peeler to create thin slices of lemongrass for garnishing.

Nutritional Values (Per 1-cup serving):

- Calories: 60

- Protein: 0g

- Fat: 0g - Carbohydrates: 15g

- Sugar: 14g - Probiotics: High

ROSEHIP AND APPLE CIDER FERMENTED TEA FOR IMMUNITY

Servings: 4 (1-cup servings)

Prep Time: 15 minutes (plus fermentation time: 2-3 days)

Ingredients:

- 4 cups water

- 1/2 cup dried rosehips

- 1/4 cup honey or agave syrup

- 1/4 cup apple cider vinegar

- 1/4 cup whey (or 2 tablespoons sea salt)

Instructions:

1. **Boil Water:** Bring water to a boil.

2. **Steep Rosehips:** Add dried rosehips to boiling water. Steep for 10 minutes, then strain and let cool.

3. **Sweeten:** Stir in honey or agave syrup and apple cider vinegar until dissolved.

4. **Add Culture:** Mix in whey or sea salt.

5. **Ferment:** Pour into a glass jar and let it ferment at room temperature for 2-3 days.

6. **Store and Serve**: Once fermented, refrigerate and serve chilled.

Tips:

- Rosehips are high in vitamin C, enhancing the immune-boosting properties.

- Consider adding a slice of fresh apple for garnish.

Nutritional Values (Per 1-cup serving):

- Calories: 70 - Protein: 0g

- Fat: 0g - Carbohydrates: 18g

- Sugar: 17g - Probiotics: High

ELDERFLOWER FERMENTED ICED TEA FOR GUT AND SKIN HEALTH

Servings: 4 (1-cup servings)

Prep Time: 15 minutes (plus fermentation time: 2-3 days)

Ingredients:

- 4 cups water

- 1/4 cup dried elderflowers

- 1/4 cup honey or agave syrup

- 1/4 cup whey (or 2 tablespoons sea salt)

- Optional: Fresh mint for garnish

Instructions:

1. **Boil Water:** Bring water to a boil.

2. **Steep Elderflowers:** Add elderflowers to boiling water and steep for 10 minutes. Strain and let cool.

3. **Sweeten:** Stir in honey or agave syrup until dissolved.

4. **Add Culture:** Mix in whey or sea salt.

5. **Ferment:** Pour into a glass jar, cover loosely, and ferment at room temperature for 2-3 days.

6. **Serve:** Once ready, strain and serve over ice.

Tips:

- Garnish with fresh mint for added freshness.

- Elderflower has anti-inflammatory properties that are beneficial for skin health.

Nutritional Values (Per 1-cup serving):

- Calories: 65

- Protein: 0g

- Fat: 0g - Carbohydrates: 17g

- Sugar: 16g - Probiotics: High

FERMENTED CHAI TEA LATTE – A WARM, SPICY PROBIOTIC DRINK

Servings: 4 (1-cup servings)

Prep Time: 15 minutes (plus fermentation time: 2-3 days)

Ingredients:

- 4 cups water

- 4 black tea bags (or 4 tablespoons loose-leaf black tea)

- 1 tablespoon chai spice blend (cinnamon, ginger, cardamom, cloves)

- 1/4 cup honey or maple syrup

- 1/4 cup whey (or 2 tablespoons sea salt)

- 1 cup milk (dairy or plant-based)

Instructions:

1. **Boil Water:** Bring water to a boil.

2. **Steep Tea and Spices:** Add tea bags and chai spices to boiling water. Steep for 10 minutes, then remove tea bags and let cool.

3. **Sweeten:** Stir in honey or maple syrup until dissolved.

4. **Add Culture:** Mix in whey or sea salt.

5. **Ferment:** Pour into a glass jar, cover loosely, and ferment at room temperature for 2-3 days.

6. **Serve:** Once ready, warm the milk and combine with the fermented chai mixture. Serve hot.

Tips:

- Adjust sweetness according to your taste.

- A sprinkle of cinnamon on top adds a lovely aroma.

Nutritional Values (Per 1-cup serving):

- Calories: 80 - Protein: 2g - Fat: 3g

- Carbohydrates: 12g - Sugar: 10g - Probiotics: High

Chapter 5

FERMENTED JUICES – SQUEEZE OUT THE GOODNESS

"Fermented juices offer a refreshing way to get a concentrated dose of probiotics while keeping your gut happy and healthy."

This chapter focuses on fruit and vegetable juices that undergo fermentation, amplifying their nutritional benefits while creating tangy, refreshing drinks. Get ready to embrace the vibrant flavors and health benefits of fermented juices that can elevate your gut health and satisfy your taste buds.

These recipes showcase the diverse and delightful ways to incorporate fermented juices into your diet, each providing a burst of flavor along with health benefits for your gut and overall wellness. Enjoy experimenting with these refreshing beverages!

FERMENTED CARROT-ORANGE JUICE FOR EYE AND GUT HEALTH

Servings: 4 (1-cup servings)

Prep Time: 15 minutes (plus fermentation time: 2-3 days)

Ingredients:

- 4 large carrots, peeled and chopped

- 2 large oranges, juiced

- 1 tablespoon grated ginger

- 1 tablespoon honey (optional)

- 1/4 cup whey (or 2 tablespoons sea salt)

- 1-2 cups filtered water (as needed)

Instructions:

1. Juice the Carrots: Use a juicer or blender to puree the carrots. If using a blender, add a little water to help blend smoothly. Strain the mixture to extract the juice.

2. Combine Juices: In a large mixing bowl, combine carrot juice, fresh orange juice, and grated ginger.

3. Sweeten (Optional): Stir in honey if desired.

4. Add Culture: Mix in whey or sea salt.

5. Ferment: Pour the mixture into a clean glass jar, leaving some space at the top for expansion. Cover loosely with a lid or cloth to allow gases to escape. Let it sit at room temperature for 2-3 days.

6. Taste Test: After fermentation, taste for tanginess. If satisfied, refrigerate the juice to slow down fermentation.

Tips:

- Adjust the sweetness by varying the amount of honey.

- Serve chilled for a refreshing drink.

Nutritional Values (Per 1-cup serving):

- Calories: 70

- Protein: 1g - Fat: 0g

- Carbohydrates: 16g - Sugar: 13g

- Probiotics: High

PINEAPPLE PAPAYA PROBIOTIC JUICE

Servings: 4 (1-cup servings)

Prep Time: 20 minutes (plus fermentation time: 2-3 days)

Ingredients:

- 2 cups fresh pineapple chunks

- 2 cups ripe papaya chunks

- 1 tablespoon grated ginger

- 1/4 cup honey (optional)

- 1/4 cup whey (or 2 tablespoons sea salt)

- 1-2 cups filtered water (as needed)

Instructions:

1. Juice Fruits: Blend pineapple and papaya in a blender until smooth. Add water as needed to reach desired consistency.

2. Combine Ingredients: Pour the juice into a mixing bowl. Stir in grated ginger and honey if using.

3. **Add Culture:** Incorporate whey or sea salt into the mixture.

4. **Ferment:** Transfer the juice to a clean glass jar, leaving space for gas expansion. Cover loosely with a lid or cloth and let ferment at room temperature for 2-3 days.

5. **Refrigerate:** Taste the juice; once tangy enough, refrigerate to halt fermentation.

Tips:

- Use ripe fruits for the best flavor.

- Add a squeeze of lime for an extra zing.

Nutritional Values (Per 1-cup serving):

- Calories: 90

- Protein: 1g - Fat: 0g

- Carbohydrates: 23g - Sugar: 20g

- Probiotics: High

FERMENTED BEET JUICE FOR DETOX AND DIGESTION

Servings: 4 (1-cup servings)

Prep Time: 15 minutes (plus fermentation time: 2-3 days)

Ingredients:

- 2 medium beets, peeled and chopped

- 1 apple, cored and chopped

- 1 tablespoon grated ginger

- 1 tablespoon honey (optional)

- 1/4 cup whey (or 2 tablespoons sea salt)

- 1-2 cups filtered water (as needed)

Instructions:

1. **Juice Beets and Apple:** Blend beets and apple together in a blender. Strain to extract juice.

2. **Mix Ingredients:** In a bowl, combine beet juice, grated ginger, and honey (if using).

3. **Add Culture:** Stir in whey or sea salt.

4. **Ferment:** Pour into a clean glass jar, cover loosely, and let ferment at room temperature for 2-3 days.

5. **Taste and Chill:** After fermentation, taste for desired tanginess, then refrigerate.

Tips:

- Beets can stain, so handle with care.

- Serve with a splash of lemon juice for added freshness.

Nutritional Values (Per 1-cup serving):

- Calories: 85

- Protein: 1g

- Fat: 0g - Carbohydrates: 20g

- Sugar: 10g - Probiotics: High

54

SPICED CRANBERRY FERMENTED JUICE – A HOLIDAY FAVORITE

Servings: 4 (1-cup servings)

Prep Time: 15 minutes (plus fermentation time: 2-3 days)

Ingredients:

- 2 cups fresh cranberries
- 1 cup apple juice (preferably fresh-pressed)
- 1 tablespoon grated ginger
- 1/4 cup honey (optional)
- 1/4 cup whey (or 2 tablespoons sea salt)
- 1-2 cups filtered water (as needed)

Instructions:

1. **Juice Cranberries:** Blend cranberries with apple juice and a little water until smooth. Strain to extract juice.

2. **Mix Ingredients:** In a bowl, combine cranberry juice, grated ginger, and honey (if desired).

3. **Add Culture:** Mix in whey or sea salt.

4. **Ferment:** Pour into a clean glass jar, cover loosely, and allow to ferment at room temperature for 2-3 days.

5. **Chill and Serve:** Once fermented to your liking, refrigerate.

Tips:

- Adjust sweetness with honey based on tartness preference.

- Use as a festive cocktail mixer.

Nutritional Values (Per 1-cup serving):

- Calories: 70 - Protein: 1g - Fat: 0g

- Carbohydrates: 17g - Sugar: 14g

- Probiotics: High

. GREEN APPLE AND SPINACH FERMENTED JUICE

Servings: 4 (1-cup servings)

Prep Time: 15 minutes (plus fermentation time: 2-3 days)

Ingredients:

- 2 green apples, cored and chopped

- 2 cups fresh spinach leaves

- 1 tablespoon lemon juice

- 1 tablespoon grated ginger

- 1/4 cup honey (optional)

- 1/4 cup whey (or 2 tablespoons sea salt)

- 1-2 cups filtered water (as needed)

Instructions:

1. **Juice Ingredients:** Blend apples, spinach, and lemon juice until smooth, adding water as needed. Strain to extract juice.

2. **Combine Juices:** In a mixing bowl, combine apple-spinach juice with grated ginger and honey (if using).

3. **Add Culture:** Stir in whey or sea salt.

4. **Ferment:** Transfer to a clean glass jar, cover loosely, and allow to ferment at room temperature for 2-3 days.

5. **Refrigerate:** Taste for tanginess, then refrigerate once ready.

Tips:

- Green apples add tartness; use sweeter apples if preferred.

- Serve over ice for a refreshing drink.

Nutritional Values (Per 1-cup serving):
Calories: 65 - Protein: 1g - Fat: 0g

- Carbohydrates: 16g - Sugar: 12g - Probiotics: H

WATERMELON FERMENTED JUICE – HYDRATION AND GUT BALANCE

Servings: 4 (1-cup servings)

Prep Time: 10 minutes (plus fermentation time: 2-3 days)

Ingredients:

- 4 cups watermelon, chopped and seeded

- 1 tablespoon lime juice

- 1/4 cup honey (optional)

- 1/4 cup whey (or 2 tablespoons sea salt)

Instructions:

1. **Juice Watermelon:** Blend watermelon chunks until smooth. Strain to extract juice.

2. **Mix Ingredients:** In a bowl, combine watermelon juice, lime juice, and honey (if using).

3. **Add Culture:** Stir in whey or sea salt.

4. **Ferment:** Pour into a clean glass jar, cover loosely, and ferment at room temperature for 2-3 days.

5. **Chill:** After fermentation, refrigerate to halt the process.

Tips:

- Watermelon juice is best served cold.

- Garnish with mint for added freshness.

Nutritional Values (Per 1-cup serving):

- Calories: 60

- Protein: 1g - Fat: 0g

- Carbohydrates: 16g

- Sugar: 14g - Probiotics: High

FERMENTED CUCUMBER-APPLE JUICE FOR COOLING DIGESTIVE RELIEF

Servings: 4 (1-cup servings)

Prep Time: 15 minutes (plus fermentation time: 2-3 days)

Ingredients:

- 2 cucumbers, peeled and chopped

- 2 green apples, cored and chopped

- 1 tablespoon lemon juice

- 1/4 cup honey (optional)

- 1/4 cup whey (or 2 tablespoons sea salt)

- 1-2 cups filtered water (as needed)

Instructions:

1. **Juice Cucumbers and Apples:** Blend cucumbers and apples until smooth, adding water as needed. Strain to extract juice.

2. **Combine Ingredients:** In a bowl, mix cucumber-apple juice with lemon juice and honey (if using).

3. **Add Culture:** Stir in whey or sea salt.

4. **Ferment:** Pour into a clean glass jar, cover loosely, and allow to ferment at room temperature for 2-3 days.

5. **Refrigerate:** Taste for tanginess, then refrigerate once desired flavor is achieved.

Tips:

- Use a mix of cucumber varieties for different flavors.

- Serve with a slice of cucumber for garnish.

Nutritional Values (Per 1-cup serving):

- Calories: 50 - Protein: 1g - Fat: 0g

- Carbohydrates: 12g - Sugar: 10g - Probiotics: High

58

LACTO-FERMENTED CARROT GINGER JUICE

Servings: 4 (1-cup servings)

Prep Time: 15 minutes (plus fermentation time: 2-3 days)

Ingredients:

- 4 large carrots, peeled and chopped

- 1 tablespoon grated ginger

- 1 tablespoon lemon juice

- 1/4 cup honey (optional)

- 1/4 cup whey (or 2 tablespoons sea salt)

- 1-2 cups filtered water (as needed)

Instructions:

1. **Juice Carrots:** Blend carrots until smooth, adding water as needed. Strain to extract juice.

2. **Combine Ingredients:** In a bowl, mix carrot juice, grated ginger, lemon juice, and honey (if using).

3. **Add Culture:** Stir in whey or sea salt.

4. **Ferment:** Pour into a clean glass jar, cover loosely, and allow to ferment at room temperature for 2-3 days.

5. **Refrigerate:** Once fermented to your liking, refrigerate.

Tips:

- Adjust ginger to taste for more or less spice.

- Perfect for sipping during cold weather.

Nutritional Values (Per 1-cup serving):

- Calories: 70

- Protein: 1g - Fat: 0g

- Carbohydrates: 16g

- Sugar: 14g - Probiotics: High

Chapter 6

FERMENTED NUT AND GRAIN MILKS – CREAMY GUT HEALERS

"Fermented nut and grain milks offer a plant-based way to enjoy creamy, probiotic-rich beverages that soothe your gut and support digestion."

Explores non-dairy milks made from almonds, oats, and rice, then fermented to enhance their probiotic content and make them a creamy, gut-friendly treat.

This chapter provides a variety of delicious and nutritious fermented nut and grain milks that not only taste great but also contribute to gut health. Enjoy exploring these creamy gut healers!

ALMOND MILK KEFIR

Servings: 4 (1-cup servings)

Prep Time: 10 minutes (plus fermentation time: 24-48 hours)

Ingredients:

- 1 cup raw almonds

- 4 cups filtered water (for soaking)

- 4 cups filtered water (for blending)

- 1/4 cup kefir grains or 1/2 cup store-bought kefir

- 1 tablespoon maple syrup or honey (optional)

- Pinch of sea salt

Instructions:

1. **Soak the Almonds:** Place the raw almonds in a bowl and cover with 4 cups of filtered water. Soak for 8-12 hours or overnight.

2. **Blend:** Drain and rinse the soaked almonds. Add them to a blender with 4 cups of filtered water. Blend on high for about 2-3 minutes until smooth and creamy.

3. **Strain:** Pour the almond mixture through a nut milk bag or fine mesh strainer into a large bowl, squeezing out as much liquid as possible. Discard the almond pulp or save it for another use.

4. **Ferment:** Transfer the almond milk to a clean glass jar and stir in the kefir grains or store-bought kefir. If desired, add maple syrup or honey for sweetness and a pinch of sea salt.

5. **Cover:** Loosely cover the jar with a clean cloth or lid to allow airflow. Let it sit at room temperature for 24-48 hours, tasting occasionally until you reach the desired tanginess.

6. **Store:** Once fermented, strain out the kefir grains (if using) and transfer the almond milk kefir to the refrigerator. Enjoy chilled.

Tips:

- Use the leftover almond pulp in smoothies or baking for added nutrition.

- For a flavored version, consider adding vanilla extract or a dash of cinnamon.

Nutritional Values (Per 1-cup serving):

- Calories: 70

- Protein: 2g - Fat: 6g

- Carbohydrates: 3g Sugar: 1g - Probiotics: High

FERMENTED OAT MILK WITH CINNAMON

Servings: 4 (1-cup servings)

Prep Time: 10 minutes (plus fermentation time: 24-48 hours)

Ingredients:

- 1 cup rolled oats

- 4 cups filtered water (for blending)

- 1/4 cup kefir grains or 1/2 cup store-bought kefir

- 1 teaspoon ground cinnamon

- 1 tablespoon maple syrup or honey (optional)

- Pinch of sea salt

Instructions:

1. **Blend Oats:** Add rolled oats and 4 cups of filtered water to a blender. Blend on high for about 30 seconds until smooth.

62

2. **Strain:** Pour the oat mixture through a nut milk bag or fine mesh strainer into a large bowl. Squeeze to extract as much liquid as possible.

3. **Ferment:** Pour the strained oat milk into a clean glass jar. Stir in the kefir grains or store-bought kefir, ground cinnamon, maple syrup or honey (if using), and a pinch of sea salt.

4. **Cover:** Loosely cover the jar and let it sit at room temperature for 24-48 hours, tasting for desired tanginess.

5. **Store:** Once fermented, strain out the kefir grains (if using) and transfer the oat milk to the refrigerator.

Tips:

- Shake well before consuming as separation may occur.

- Enjoy this oat milk in smoothies, coffee, or as a standalone beverage.

Nutritional Values (Per 1-cup serving):

- Calories: 80

- Protein: 3g

- Fat: 2g - Carbohydrates: 14g

- Sugar: 2g - Probiotics: High

CASHEW MILK KEFIR SMOOTHIE WITH BERRIES

Servings: 2 (1-cup servings)

Prep Time: 15 minutes (plus fermentation time: 24 hours)

Ingredients:

- 1 cup raw cashews

- 4 cups filtered water (for blending)

- 1/4 cup kefir grains or 1/2 cup store-bought kefir

- 1 cup mixed berries (fresh or frozen)

- 1 tablespoon maple syrup or honey (optional)

- 1 teaspoon vanilla extract

- Pinch of sea salt

Instructions:

1. **Soak Cashews:** Soak the raw cashews in 4 cups of water for 4-6 hours. Drain and rinse.

2. **Blend:** In a blender, combine soaked cashews and 4 cups of fresh filtered water. Blend on high until smooth and creamy.

3. **Ferment:** Pour the cashew milk into a clean glass jar and stir in the kefir grains or store-bought kefir. If desired, add maple syrup, vanilla extract, and a pinch of sea salt.

4. **Cover:** Loosely cover the jar and let it sit at room temperature for 24 hours to ferment.

5. **Smoothie Preparation:** After fermentation, blend the cashew milk with mixed berries until smooth. Serve chilled.

Tips:

- For added thickness, blend in a banana or additional frozen berries. - This smoothie can be a perfect breakfast or snack option.

Nutritional Values (Per 1-cup serving):

- Calories: 120 - Protein: 4g

- Fat: 8g - Carbohydrates: 10g

- Sugar: 3g - Probiotics: High

RICE MILK KEFIR FOR DAIRY-FREE GUT HEALING

Servings: 4 (1-cup servings)

Prep Time: 10 minutes (plus fermentation time: 24-48 hours)

Ingredients:

- 1 cup uncooked white or brown rice

- 4 cups filtered water (for blending)

- 1/4 cup kefir grains or 1/2 cup store-bought kefir

- 1 tablespoon maple syrup or honey (optional)

- Pinch of sea salt

Instructions:

1. **Cook Rice:** Rinse the rice under cold water. Cook it according to package instructions.

2. **Blend:** Once cooked and cooled, add the rice to a blender with 4 cups of filtered water. Blend until smooth and creamy.

3. **Strain:** Pour the rice milk through a nut milk bag or fine mesh strainer into a large bowl. Squeeze out as much liquid as possible.

4. **Ferment:** Transfer the rice milk to a clean glass jar and stir in the kefir grains or store-bought kefir, along with maple syrup and sea salt if using.

5. **Cover:** Loosely cover and let it ferment at room temperature for 24-48 hours.

6. **Store:** Once fermented, strain out the kefir grains and store the rice milk in the refrigerator.

Tips:

- Use this rice milk in smoothies, baking, or as a base for soups. - Enhance flavor with a touch of vanilla or cinnamon if desired.

Nutritional Values (Per 1-cup serving):

- Calories: 90 - Protein: 2g - Fat: 2g

- Carbohydrates: 19g - Sugar: 0g

- Probiotics: High

HAZELNUT MILK KEFIR WITH CACAO NIBS – A DECADENT PROBIOTIC TREAT

Servings: 4 (1-cup servings)

Prep Time: 10 minutes (plus fermentation time: 24-48 hours)

Ingredients:

- 1 cup raw hazelnuts

- 4 cups filtered water (for blending)

- 1/4 cup kefir grains or 1/2 cup store-bought kefir

- 1 tablespoon cacao nibs

- 1 tablespoon maple syrup or honey (optional)

- Pinch of sea salt

Instructions:

1. **Soak Hazelnuts:** Soak the raw hazelnuts in 4 cups of water for 8-12 hours. Drain and rinse.

2. **Blend:** Combine soaked hazelnuts with 4 cups of fresh filtered water in a blender. Blend until smooth and creamy.

3. **Strain:** Strain the mixture through a nut milk bag or fine mesh strainer into a bowl, squeezing out as much liquid as possible.

4. **Ferment:** Pour the hazelnut milk into a clean glass jar. Stir in the kefir grains or store-bought kefir, cacao nibs, maple syrup (if using), and sea salt.

5. **Cover:** Loosely cover and let it sit at room temperature for 24-48 hours.

6. **Store:** Once fermented, strain out the kefir grains and cacao nibs, then refrigerate the hazelnut milk.

- Serve chilled over ice or as a base for smoothies.

- For extra indulgence, blend in additional cacao nibs just before serving.

Nutritional Values (Per 1-cup serving):

- Calories: 100

- Protein: 3g - Fat: 6g

- Carbohydrates: 10g - Sugar: 2g

- Probiotics: High

FERMENTED COCONUT MILK LATTE

Servings: 2 (1-cup servings)

Prep Time: 10 minutes (plus fermentation time: 24 hours)

Ingredients:

- 2 cups canned coconut milk

- 2 cups filtered water

- 1/4 cup kefir grains or 1/2 cup store-bought kefir

- 1 tablespoon maple syrup or honey (optional)

- 1 teaspoon vanilla extract

- Pinch of sea salt

- 1-2 shots of espresso or strong coffee (optional)

Instructions:

1. **Combine Ingredients:** In a bowl, mix the canned coconut milk with 2 cups of filtered water until well combined.

2. **Ferment:** Pour the mixture into a clean glass jar and stir in the kefir grains or store-bought kefir. Add maple syrup, vanilla extract, and sea salt if using.

3. **Cover:** Loosely cover the jar and let it sit at room temperature for 24 hours to ferment.

4. **Prepare Latte:** After fermentation, stir the coconut milk kefir into freshly brewed espresso or strong coffee. Serve hot or iced.

Tips:

- For a frothy texture, use a milk frother before adding to coffee.

- Top with a sprinkle of cinnamon or cocoa powder for extra flavor.

Nutritional Values (Per 1-cup serving, without coffee):

- Calories: 160

- Protein: 2g - Fat: 15g

- Carbohydrates: 6g - Sugar: 2g

- Probiotics: High

MACADAMIA NUT MILK KEFIR FOR LUXURIOUS CREAMINESS

Servings: 4 (1-cup servings)

Prep Time: 10 minutes (plus fermentation time: 24-48 hours)

Ingredients:

- 1 cup raw macadamia nuts

- 4 cups filtered water (for blending)

- 1/4 cup kefir grains or 1/2 cup store-bought kefir

- 1 tablespoon maple syrup or honey (optional)

- Pinch of sea salt

Instructions:

1. **Soak Macadamia Nuts:** Soak the macadamia nuts in water for 4-6 hours. Drain and rinse.

2. **Blend:** Combine the soaked nuts with 4 cups of filtered water in a blender and blend until smooth.

3. **Strain:** Strain the mixture through a nut milk bag or fine mesh strainer into a bowl, squeezing to extract as much liquid as possible.

4. **Ferment:** Pour the macadamia milk into a clean glass jar. Stir in kefir grains or store-bought kefir, adding maple syrup and a pinch of sea salt if desired.

5. **Cover:** Loosely cover and let it ferment at room temperature for 24-48 hours.

6. **Store:** Once fermented, strain out the kefir grains and refrigerate the macadamia milk.

Tips:

- This milk is particularly rich and can be used in desserts or as a coffee creamer.

- Experiment with flavorings like vanilla or almond extract.

Nutritional Values (Per 1-cup serving):

- Calories: 200 - Protein: 2g

- Fat: 21g - Carbohydrates: 6g

- Sugar: 2g - Probiotics: High

FERMENTED QUINOA MILK WITH VANILLA

Servings: 4 (1-cup servings)

Prep Time: 10 minutes (plus fermentation time: 24-48 hours)

Ingredients:

- 1 cup cooked quinoa

- 4 cups filtered water (for blending)

- 1/4 cup kefir grains or 1/2 cup store-bought kefir

- 1 tablespoon maple syrup or honey (optional)

- 1 teaspoon vanilla extract

- Pinch of sea salt

Instructions:

1. **Cook Quinoa:** Rinse and cook the quinoa according to package instructions. Allow it to cool.

2. **Blend:** In a blender, combine cooked quinoa and 4 cups of filtered water. Blend until smooth.

3. **Strain:** Strain the mixture through a nut milk bag or fine mesh strainer into a large bowl.

4. **Ferment:** Transfer the quinoa milk to a clean glass jar and stir in kefir grains or store-bought kefir, along with maple syrup, vanilla extract, and sea salt if desired.

5. **Cover:** Loosely cover the jar and let it ferment at room temperature for 24-48 hours.

6. **Store:** Once fermented, strain out the kefir grains and refrigerate the quinoa milk.

Tips:

- This milk can be enjoyed in smoothies, coffee, or used in baking.

- For extra flavor, try adding a pinch of cinnamon or nutmeg.

Nutritional Values (Per 1-cup serving):

- Calories: 110

- Protein: 4g - Fat: 2g

- Carbohydrates: 20g

- Sugar: 2g - Probiotics: High

Chapter 7

FERMENTED SMOOTHIES – BLENDING FLAVOR AND GUT HEALTH

"Imagine starting your day with a smoothie that not only tastes great but also floods your gut with beneficial bacteria."

In this chapter, you'll discover how to incorporate fermented fruits, vegetables, and kefirs into creative smoothie recipes that are loaded with probiotics and flavor.

These fermented smoothies not only tantalize your taste buds but also support gut health with their probiotic-rich ingredients. Enjoy experimenting with these recipes and the benefits they bring to your well-being!

TROPICAL FERMENTED PINEAPPLE-COCONUT SMOOTHIE

Servings: 2

Prep Time: 10 minutes (plus fermentation time: 12-24 hours)

Ingredients:

- 1 cup fresh pineapple chunks (or canned pineapple in juice)

- 1 cup canned coconut milk

- 1/2 cup plain kefir (or coconut kefir)

- 1 tablespoon honey or maple syrup (optional)

- 1/2 teaspoon vanilla extract

- 1/2 cup ice cubes

Instructions:

1. **Prepare Pineapple:** If using fresh pineapple, peel and chop it into chunks. If using canned, drain the pineapple.

2. **Blend Ingredients:** In a blender, combine the pineapple, coconut milk, kefir, honey or maple syrup, vanilla extract, and ice cubes. Blend until smooth.

3. **Ferment:** Pour the smoothie into a clean glass jar, cover it loosely, and let it sit at room temperature for 12-24 hours to ferment. The longer it ferments, the tangier it will taste.

4. **Chill and Serve:** After fermentation, refrigerate the smoothie for at least an hour before serving. Stir well and pour into glasses.

Tips:

- Adjust the sweetness to your taste by adding more or less honey/maple syrup. - For a tropical twist, add a few slices of banana or mango before blending.

Nutritional Values (Per serving):

- Calories: 200 - Protein: 4g

- Fat: 9g - Carbohydrates: 28g

- Sugar: 12g - Probiotics: High

FERMENTED BLUEBERRY OAT SMOOTHIE FOR BREAKFAST ON THE GO

Servings: 2

Prep Time: 5 minutes (plus fermentation time: 12-24 hours)

Ingredients:

- 1 cup frozen blueberries

- 1/2 cup rolled oats

- 1 cup plain yogurt (or dairy-free yogurt)

- 1 cup almond milk

- 1 tablespoon chia seeds

- 1 tablespoon honey or agave syrup (optional)

Instructions:

1. Combine Ingredients: In a blender, add frozen blueberries, rolled oats, yogurt, almond milk, chia seeds, and honey or agave syrup. Blend until smooth.

2. Ferment: Pour the smoothie into a clean glass jar, cover loosely, and let it ferment at room temperature for 12-24 hours.

3. Serve: Once fermented, stir well and pour into two glasses. Enjoy immediately.

Tips:

- For a creamier texture, use Greek yogurt.

- Add a handful of spinach for extra nutrients without altering the flavor.

Nutritional Values (Per serving):

- Calories: 220

- Protein: 8g - Fat: 6g

- Carbohydrates: 36g

- Sugar: 10g - Probiotics: Moderate

GREEN GUT BOOSTER SMOOTHIE WITH SPINACH AND KOMBUCHA

Servings: 2

Prep Time: 10 minutes

Ingredients:

- 1 cup fresh spinach
- 1/2 avocado
- 1 cup kombucha (any flavor)
- 1 banana
- 1 tablespoon flaxseeds
- 1 tablespoon lemon juice
- Ice cubes (optional)

Instructions:

1. **Blend Ingredients:** In a blender, combine spinach, avocado, kombucha, banana, flaxseeds, and lemon juice. Blend until smooth and creamy. Add ice cubes if desired.

2. **Serve:** Pour into glasses and enjoy immediately.

Tips:

- Choose a citrus-flavored kombucha for a refreshing twist.

- Add a scoop of protein powder for an extra nutritional boost.

Nutritional Values (Per serving):

- Calories: 180

- Protein: 4g

- Fat: 9g

- Carbohydrates: 26g

- Sugar: 10g

- Probiotics: High

. FERMENTED MANGO-BANANA SMOOTHIE

Servings: 2

Prep Time: 10 minutes (plus fermentation time: 12-24 hours)

Ingredients:

- 1 ripe mango, peeled and diced
- 1 ripe banana
- 1 cup coconut yogurt (or dairy-free yogurt)
- 1/2 cup orange juice
- 1 tablespoon ginger (grated)
- 1 tablespoon honey (optional)

Instructions:

1. **Blend Ingredients:** In a blender, add mango, banana, coconut yogurt, orange juice, ginger, and honey. Blend until smooth.

2. **Ferment:** Pour into a clean glass jar, cover loosely, and let it ferment at room temperature for 12-24 hours.

3. **Serve:** After fermentation, refrigerate and stir before serving.

Tips:

- For a spicier kick, add a pinch of cayenne pepper.

- Garnish with a sprinkle of shredded coconut for added texture.

Nutritional Values (Per serving):

- Calories: 210

- Protein: 5g - Fat: 4g

- Carbohydrates: 45g

- Sugar: 20g - Probiotics: Moderate

STRAWBERRY KEFIR SMOOTHIE WITH FLAXSEED

Servings: 2

Prep Time: 10 minutes

Ingredients:

- 1 cup fresh or frozen strawberries

- 1 cup plain kefir

- 1 tablespoon flaxseed meal

- 1 tablespoon honey or maple syrup (optional)

- 1/2 cup almond milk (adjust for desired consistency)

Instructions:

1. Blend Ingredients: In a blender, combine strawberries, kefir, flaxseed meal, honey, and almond milk. Blend until smooth.

2. Serve: Pour into glasses and enjoy immediately.

Tips:

- Substitute strawberries with any berry of your choice for a different flavor.

- Add a handful of spinach for extra nutrients without changing the taste.

Nutritional Values (Per serving):

- Calories: 150

- Protein: 6g - Fat: 3g

- Carbohydrates: 24g - Sugar: 10g

- Probiotics: High

FERMENTED CARROT-ORANGE GINGER SMOOTHIE

Servings: 2

Prep Time: 10 minutes (plus fermentation time: 12-24 hours)

Ingredients:

- 1 cup fresh carrots, chopped

- 1 orange, peeled and segmented

- 1 tablespoon fresh ginger (grated)

- 1 cup plain yogurt (or non-dairy yogurt)

- 1 tablespoon honey (optional)

- 1/2 cup water (adjust for desired consistency)

Instructions:

1. Blend Ingredients: In a blender, combine carrots, orange, ginger, yogurt, honey, and water. Blend until smooth.

2. Ferment: Pour into a clean glass jar, cover loosely, and let it ferment at room temperature for 12-24 hours.

3. Serve: Refrigerate and stir before serving.

Tips:

- Add a pinch of turmeric for extra health benefits and a beautiful color.

- Serve chilled for a refreshing drink on a hot day.

Nutritional Values (Per serving):

- Calories: 180

- Protein: 5g - Fat: 3g

- Carbohydrates: 37g

- Sugar: 12g - Probiotics: Moderate

BEET AND APPLE FERMENTED POWER SMOOTHIE

Servings: 2

Prep Time: 10 minutes (plus fermentation time: 12-24 hours)

Ingredients:

- 1 medium beet, cooked and chopped

- 1 apple, cored and diced

- 1 cup plain kefir

- 1 tablespoon lemon juice

- 1 tablespoon maple syrup (optional)

- 1/2 cup water (adjust for desired consistency)

Instructions:

1. Blend Ingredients: In a blender, combine beet, apple, kefir, lemon juice, maple syrup, and water. Blend until smooth.

2. Ferment: Pour into a clean glass jar, cover loosely, and let it ferment at room temperature for 12-24 hours.

3. Serve: Refrigerate and stir well before serving.

Tips:

- Garnish with chopped nuts or seeds for added texture and nutrition.

- Add a pinch of cinnamon for a warm flavor.

Nutritional Values (Per serving):

- Calories: 160

- Protein: 5g

- Fat: 2g - Carbohydrates: 30g

- Sugar: 12g - Probiotics: High

. FERMENTED AVOCADO CUCUMBER SMOOTHIE FOR GUT HYDRATION

Servings: 2

Prep Time: 10 minutes

Ingredients:

- 1 ripe avocado

- 1/2 cucumber, peeled and chopped

- 1 cup coconut water

- 1/2 cup plain kefir

- 1 tablespoon lime juice

- Pinch of sea salt

- Ice cubes (optional)

Instructions:

1. **Blend Ingredients:** In a blender, combine avocado, cucumber, coconut water, kefir, lime juice, and sea salt. Blend until smooth and creamy.

2. **Serve:** Pour into glasses and enjoy immediately. Add ice cubes if desired.

Tips:

- For extra creaminess, add a handful of spinach.

- Garnish with cucumber slices for a refreshing touch.

Nutritional Values (Per serving):

- Calories: 210

- Protein: 6g - Fat: 12g

- Carbohydrates: 22g

- Sugar: 4g - Probiotics: High

Chapter 8

ALCOHOL-FREE FERMENTED 'MOCKTAILS' – GUT-FRIENDLY PARTY DRINKS

"Who says you need alcohol to have fun? These fermented mocktails pack a probiotic punch, giving you great taste and gut health benefits without the booze."

This chapter focuses on alcohol-free fermented beverages that resemble cocktails, perfect for social occasions where you want to enjoy a flavorful drink while taking care of your gut.

These alcohol-free fermented 'mocktails' not only deliver a delightful taste experience but also support gut health with their probiotic-rich ingredients. Enjoy these refreshing beverages at your next gathering!

FERMENTED GINGER MOJITO MOCKTAIL

Servings: 2

Prep Time: 10 minutes (plus fermentation time: 12-24 hours)

Ingredients:

- 1 cup fresh mint leaves, packed
- 1/4 cup fresh ginger, grated
- 1/4 cup honey or agave syrup
- 2 cups sparkling water
- Juice of 2 limes
- Ice cubes
- Extra mint leaves and lime wedges for garnish

Instructions:

1. **Make the Base:** In a bowl, combine the grated ginger, mint leaves, and honey. Use a muddler or the back of a spoon to crush the ingredients gently, releasing the mint oils and ginger juice.

2. **Add Lime Juice:** Stir in the lime juice until combined.

3. **Ferment:** Transfer the mixture to a clean glass jar, cover loosely, and let it ferment at room temperature for 12-24 hours.

4. **Mix with Sparkling Water:** After fermentation, strain the mixture into a pitcher, discarding the solids. Add the sparkling water and stir well.

5. **Serve:** Pour over ice and garnish with mint leaves and lime wedges.

Tips:

- For a stronger ginger flavor, add more grated ginger before fermentation.

- If you prefer a sweeter drink, adjust the honey or agave syrup to taste.

Nutritional Values (Per serving):

- Calories: 90

- Protein: 1g - Fat: 0g

- Carbohydrates: 23g - Sugar: 19g

- Probiotics: Moderate

KOMBUCHA SANGRIA WITH FERMENTED FRUIT

Servings: 4

Prep Time: 15 minutes (plus fermentation time: 12-24 hours)

Ingredients:

- 2 cups mixed berries (strawberries, blueberries, raspberries)

- 1 cup diced peaches or nectarines

- 1 bottle (16 oz) kombucha (preferably berry-flavored)

- 1 cup orange juice

- 1/2 cup club soda

- 1 tablespoon honey or agave syrup (optional)

- Fresh mint for garnish

Instructions:

1. **Prepare the Fruit:** In a large pitcher, combine mixed berries and diced peaches. Add honey or agave syrup if desired and gently muddle the fruit to release juices.

2. **Add Kombucha and Orange Juice:** Pour in the kombucha and orange juice. Stir gently to combine.

3. **Ferment:** Cover the pitcher loosely and let it sit at room temperature for 12-24 hours to ferment slightly.

4. **Finish and Serve:** Stir in the club soda just before serving. Pour into glasses over ice and garnish with fresh mint.

Tips:

- Feel free to use any seasonal fruits you have on hand.

- For a more refreshing drink, add a splash of lemon or lime juice.

Nutritional Values (Per serving):

- Calories: 80 - Protein: 1g

- Fat: 0g - Carbohydrates: 19g

- Sugar: 15g

- Probiotics: High

LACTO-FERMENTED WATERMELON MARGARITA

Servings: 2

Prep Time: 10 minutes (plus fermentation time: 12-24 hours)

Ingredients:

- 2 cups seedless watermelon, cubed

- 1/4 cup lime juice

- 1 tablespoon honey or agave syrup (optional)

- 1/2 cup plain yogurt or coconut yogurt

- 1/4 cup sparkling water

- Lime slices and watermelon wedges for garnish

- Ice cubes

Instructions:

1. **Blend the Watermelon**: In a blender, puree the watermelon until smooth. Strain the juice into a bowl, discarding the pulp.

2. **Mix Ingredients**: Combine the watermelon juice, lime juice, yogurt, and honey/agave syrup in a jar and stir well.

3. **Ferment**: Cover the jar loosely and let it sit at room temperature for 12-24 hours.

4. **Serve**: After fermentation, mix in the sparkling water. Pour over ice and garnish with lime slices and watermelon wedges.

Tips:

- Use a melon baller to create decorative watermelon balls for garnishing.

- For an added zing, consider adding a pinch of sea salt.

Nutritional Values (Per serving):

- Calories: 120

- Protein: 4g

- Fat: 2g - Carbohydrates: 24g

- Sugar: 18g - Probiotics: M

CUCUMBER BASIL KEFIR COLLINS

Servings: 2

Prep Time: 10 minutes (plus fermentation time: 12-24 hours)

Ingredients:

- 1 cup cucumber, peeled and sliced

- 1/4 cup fresh basil leaves

- 1 cup plain kefir

- Juice of 1 lemon

- 1 tablespoon honey or agave syrup (optional)

- 1 cup sparkling water

- Ice cubes

- Basil sprigs and cucumber slices for garnish

Instructions:

1. **Blend Cucumber and Basil:** In a blender, combine cucumber slices, basil leaves, lemon juice, and honey/agave syrup. Blend until smooth.

2. **Mix with Kefir:** Add the kefir and blend again until well combined.

3. **Ferment:** Pour the mixture into a clean jar, cover loosely, and let it ferment for 12-24 hours.

4. **Serve:** After fermentation, stir in the sparkling water. Pour over ice and garnish with basil sprigs and cucumber slices.

Tips:

- For a stronger basil flavor, add more fresh basil leaves before blending.

- Use flavored sparkling water for an extra burst of flavor.

Nutritional Values (Per serving):

- Calories: 90 - Protein: 5g - Fat: 2g

- Carbohydrates: 16g - Sugar: 10g

- Probiotics: High

SPICY FERMENTED BLOODY MARY

Servings: 2

Prep Time: 10 minutes (plus fermentation time: 12-24 hours)

Ingredients:

- 2 cups tomato juice (preferably homemade)

- 1/4 cup lemon juice

- 1 tablespoon Worcestershire sauce

- 1 teaspoon hot sauce (adjust to taste)

- 1 tablespoon horseradish (optional)

- 1/2 cup plain kefir

- Celery sticks and lemon wedges for garnish

- Salt and pepper to taste

Instructions:

1. **Combine Ingredients:** In a mixing bowl, whisk together the tomato juice, lemon juice, Worcestershire sauce, hot sauce, horseradish, salt, and pepper.

2. **Add Kefir:** Stir in the kefir until well combined.

3. **Ferment:** Pour the mixture into a clean glass jar, cover loosely, and let it ferment for 12-24 hours.

4. **Serve:** After fermentation, stir well and serve over ice, garnished with celery sticks and lemon wedges.

Tips:

- For an extra kick, add more hot sauce or a pinch of cayenne pepper.

- Garnish with pickles or olives for a classic Bloody Mary touch.

Nutritional Values (Per serving):

- Calories: 120 - Protein: 5g

- Fat: 3g - Carbohydrates: 20g

- Sugar: 8g - Probiotics: High

SPARKLING LAVENDER LEMONADE MOCKTAIL

Servings: 4

Prep Time: 10 minutes (plus fermentation time: 12-24 hours)

Ingredients:

- 1 cup fresh lemon juice

- 1/2 cup honey or agave syrup

- 2 cups water

- 2 tablespoons dried lavender flowers

- 2 cups sparkling water

- Lemon slices and lavender sprigs for garnish

- Ice cubes

Instructions:

1. **Make Lavender Syrup:** In a saucepan, combine water and dried lavender flowers. Bring to a boil, then reduce heat and simmer for 5 minutes. Strain the lavender and let the syrup cool.

2. **Mix Lemonade:** In a pitcher, combine fresh lemon juice, lavender syrup, and honey/agave syrup. Stir until well mixed.

3. **Ferment:** Pour the mixture into a clean glass jar, cover loosely, and let it ferment for 12-24 hours

4. **Serve:** After fermentation, stir in sparkling water. Pour over ice and garnish with lemon slices and lavender sprigs.

Tips:

- Adjust the sweetness by adding more or less honey/agave syrup.

- For an elegant touch, freeze lavender flowers in ice cubes and use them for serving.

Nutritional Values (Per serving):

- Calories: 80 - Protein: 1g

- Fat: 0g

- Carbohydrates: 20g

- Sugar: 15g - Probiotics: Moderate

CRANBERRY-ORANGE KOMBUCHA MIMOSA

Servings: 2

Prep Time: 5 minutes

Ingredients:

- 1 cup cranberry juice (unsweetened)

- 1 cup orange juice

- 2 cups kombucha (plain or orange-flavored)

- Fresh cranberries and orange slices for garnish

- Ice cubes (optional)

Instructions:

1. **Combine Juices:** In a pitcher, mix cranberry juice and orange juice until well combined.

2. **Add Kombucha:** Slowly pour in the kombucha to preserve its fizz. Stir gently to mix.

3. **Serve:** Pour into glasses over ice (if desired) and garnish with fresh cranberries and orange slices.

Tips:

- Choose a cranberry juice with no added sugar for a healthier option.

- For a festive touch, rim glasses with sugar before serving.

Nutritional Values (Per serving):

- Calories: 60

- Protein: 1g

- Fat: 0g - Carbohydrates: 15g

- Sugar: 10g

- Probiotics: High

LACTO-FERMENTED POMEGRANATE PUNCH

Servings: 4

Prep Time: 10 minutes (plus fermentation time: 12-24 hours)

Ingredients:

- 2 cups pomegranate juice (unsweetened)

- 1 cup orange juice

- 1/4 cup honey or agave syrup (optional)

- 1 cup plain yogurt or coconut yogurt

- 2 cups sparkling water

- Pomegranate seeds and orange slices for garnish

- Ice cubes

Instructions:

1. **Combine Juices:** In a bowl, mix pomegranate juice, orange juice, and honey/agave syrup until combined.

2. **Add Yogurt:** Stir in the yogurt until smooth.

3. **Ferment:** Pour the mixture into a clean glass jar, cover loosely, and let it ferment for 12-24 hours.

4. **Serve:** After fermentation, mix in the sparkling water. Pour over ice and garnish with pomegranate seeds and orange slices.

Tips:

- To intensify the flavor, consider adding a splash of lime juice.

- For a fun presentation, serve in clear glasses to showcase the vibrant color.

Nutritional Values (Per serving):

- Calories: 120 - Protein: 5g

- Fat: 2g - Carbohydrates: 25g

- Sugar: 18g - Probiotics: High